ENLARGEMENT OF THE PENIS

ways and methods men should do to last longer in bed

Dr. John K. Moore

We would be grateful if you could a few moments after you have finished reading, to please leave us a pleasing review on Amazon. Your review will help us to reach a wider audience and also help other readers to discover how helpful this book is.

Your time is valued as you are willing to share your thoughts.

Thank you in anticipation for the kind review.

Table of Contents

Dr. John K. Moore

Chapter 1

Cannutopia

Cannutopia CBD Gummies - Every man wants a performance that is steady and lasts for a long time. Unfortunately, the natural process of aging has a detrimental effect on their sexual well-being, causing individuals to become sexually depressed and feeble as they become older. As a consequence of this, individuals grow weary both physically and sexually to give their best performance, and as a result, they look for vitamins that are both healthy and effective to recover their sexual well-being. Cannutopia CBD Gummies are chewable candies that are made entirely of natural ingredients and have a high concentration of cannabidiol. They are formulated to enhance sexual health and performance in the bedroom.

Cannutopia CBD Gummies are a completely natural treatment for sexual dysfunction because they improve both performance and excitability when you're in the bedroom.

The combination stimulates the body's synthesis of testosterone, which not only restores a healthy sexual equilibrium but also boosts endurance and stamina for sustained physical activity. The gummies are also helpful in boosting good blood circulation, which contributes to the development of erections that are more stable and last for a longer period.

Cannutopia CBD Gummies are all-natural male enhancement gummies that assist men to increase their performance in the bedroom. Cannutopia CBD Gummies contain no artificial ingredients. CBD gummies provide the most effective form of support for males.

After utilizing it for a short period, you will be able to fully understand the benefits of this male enhancement medication. If you're having trouble getting an erection, try using the CBD solution. This male enhancement gummy solution can help you fulfill the woman you love more than ever before.

The candies can even enable you to boost the intensity of your orgasms and provide your partner with more satisfying erections that are more robust and larger in circumference. Consuming the gummies in the quantities that are recommended is necessary to achieve satisfying sexual benefits.

Users are always interested in learning about the operation of the supplement before they consume the gummies. According to the findings of the research and analysis that we conducted, the gummies work in a way that is completely natural to restore both your health and your sexual performance. The gummies are made up of a healthy and powerful blend of herbs and clinically approved ingredients. This combination works in a special way to restore your sexual well-being and performance while preventing age-related declines in sexual desire and exhaustion.

The goal of these candies is to increase and restore the body's natural testosterone production. It is the male support hormone that contributes to the regulation of both an individual's physical performance and endurance, as well as their sexual well-being and endurance.

As a consequence of this, it not only helps you achieve higher levels of arousal and sexual drive, but it also lessens the exhaustion and age-related declines that come along with them.

What Kinds of Ingredients Can Be Found in Cannutopia's CBD Gummies?

Extract of Tribulus Terrestris: This is a botanical component that has been shown in clinical studies to enhance healthy testosterone levels in the body. Tribulus terrestris extract. It helps to stimulate the production of the luteinizing hormone as well as enhance testosterone levels in the body, both of which are necessary for healthy biological functioning and control. It also makes your erections harder and makes you physically and sexually stronger, which enables you to perform better when you're in the bedroom.

L-Arginine is a molecule that plays a role in the stimulation of your body's levels of nitric oxide as well as the increase in blood circulation that results from this stimulation. The increased flow of blood contributes to the healthy operation of the gentile region of the body.

It assists in making your erections harder and longer, and it also helps expand the size and girth of your penis when you are engaging in sexual activity. Even erectile dysfunction (ED) and premature ejaculations can be helped by it.

Saw Palmetto Berry Extract: This is a fruit extract that has been proven to increase levels of testosterone and improve sexual health. It helps to improve sexual cravings and libido levels, as well as sexual stamina, which enables you to perform for extended periods without being exhausted. In addition to this, it supplies your body with vital nutrients, which not only increase your libido but also your sexual drive.

This chemical helps in the natural treatment of erectile dysfunction while also enhancing sexual drive and the rate of male fertility. Eurycoma Longifolia Extract is a good example of this chemical. Additionally, there is evidence that it helps men perform better in sporting events. It does this by reducing the number of fat cells throughout the body while simultaneously enhancing the development of muscle.

Dr. John K. Moore

Is purchasing Cannutopia CBD Gummies a waste of money or not?

Cannutopia CBD Gummies - Every man wants a performance that is steady and lasts for a long time. Unfortunately, the natural process of aging has a detrimental effect on their sexual well-being, causing individuals to become sexually depressed and feeble as they become older. As a consequence of this, individuals grow weary both physically and sexually to give their best performance, and as a result, they look for vitamins that are both healthy and effective to recover their sexual well-being. Cannutopia CBD Gummies are chewable candies that are made entirely of natural ingredients and have a high concentration of cannabidiol.

They are formulated to enhance sexual health and performance in the bedroom. Cannutopia CBD Gummies are a completely natural treatment for sexual dysfunction because they improve both performance and excitability when you're in the bedroom. The combination stimulates the body's synthesis of testosterone, which not only restores a healthy sexual equilibrium but also boosts endurance and stamina for sustained physical activity.

The gummies are also helpful in boosting good blood circulation, which contributes to the development of erections that are more stable and last for a longer period.

Cannutopia CBD Gummies are all-natural male enhancement gummies that assist men to increase their performance in the bedroom. Cannutopia CBD Gummies contain no artificial ingredients. CBD gummies provide the most effective form of support for males. These reviews of Cannutopia CBD Gummies are essential to addressing and advancing issues that pertain to men's health. Any male can start performing right away and have little to no difficulty doing so.

After utilizing it for a short period, you will be able to fully understand the benefits of this male enhancement medication. If you're having trouble getting an erection, try using the CBD solution. This male enhancement gummy solution can help you fulfill the woman you love more than ever before. The candies can even enable you to boost the intensity of your orgasms and provide your partner with more satisfying erections that are more robust and larger in circumference.

Consuming the gummies in the quantities that are recommended is necessary to achieve satisfying sexual benefits.

Users are always interested in learning about the operation of the supplement before they consume the gummies. According to the findings of the research and analysis that we conducted, the gummies work in a way that is completely natural to restore both your health and your sexual performance. The gummies are made up of a healthy and powerful blend of herbs and clinically approved ingredients.

This combination works in a special way to restore your sexual well-being and performance while preventing age-related declines in sexual desire and exhaustion. The goal of these candies is to increase and restore the body's natural testosterone production. It is the male support hormone that contributes to the regulation of both an individual's physical performance and endurance, as well as their sexual well-being and endurance.

As a consequence of this, it not only helps you achieve higher levels of arousal and sexual drive, but it also lessens the exhaustion and age-related declines that come along with them.

What Kinds of Ingredients Can Be Found in Cannutopia's CBD Gummies?

Tribulus Terrestris Extract: This is a component made from herbs that have been demonstrated in controlled medical studies to increase the levels of healthy testosterone in the body. It helps to stimulate the production of the luteinizing hormone as well as enhance testosterone levels in the body, both of which are necessary for healthy biological functioning and control. It also makes your erections harder and makes you physically and sexually stronger, which enables you to perform better when you're in the bedroom.

L-Arginine is a molecule that plays a role in the stimulation of your body's levels of nitric oxide as well as the increase in blood circulation that results from this stimulation. The increased flow of blood contributes to the healthy operation of the gentile region of the body.

It assists in making your erections harder and longer, and it also helps expand the size and girth of your penis when you are engaging in sexual activity. Even erectile dysfunction (ED) and premature ejaculations can be helped by it.

Saw Palmetto Berry Extract: This is a fruit extract that has been proven to increase levels of testosterone and improve sexual health.

It helps to improve sexual cravings and libido levels, as well as sexual stamina, which enables you to perform for extended periods without being exhausted. In addition to this, it supplies your body with vital nutrients, which not only increase your libido but also your sexual drive.

This chemical helps in the natural treatment of erectile dysfunction while also enhancing sexual drive and the rate of male fertility. Eurycoma Longifolia Extract is a good example of this chemical. Additionally, there is evidence that it helps men perform better in sporting events. It does this by reducing the number of fat cells throughout the body while simultaneously enhancing the development of muscle.

The Research That Supports the Claims Made by Cannutopia's CBD Gummies

Cannutopia CBD Gummies are a libido enhancer that assists persons who have experienced sexual dysfunction in regaining their previous level of sexual potency. It makes use of herbs and nutrients that have been shown in multiple studies to increase sex drive and stamina, as well as lean muscle mass and a reduction in performance anxiety.

The added feature accommodates a divers of ingredients, one of which is called Eurycoma Longifolia.

Chapter 2

Foods and Fruits That Can Enlarge Your Penis

It is becoming more common for younger men to experience erectile dysfunction, and around one in eight men may acquire prostate cancer at some point throughout their lives; hence, your sexual health and prostate health may be at the forefront of your thoughts. Diet may, surprisingly, be one of the unanticipated means by which one might improve their sexual health. Your body, including your genitalia and the rest of your sexual organs, gets the fundamental components—the building blocks—it needs to function properly from the food that you eat.

However, rather than eating as if your penis requires special attention, you can fill your day with nutritious whole foods that help your blood deliver the nutrients that your penis, prostate, and other sexual organs require to function at their absolute best. This will help you avoid eating as if your penis requires special attention.

These foods may help enhance your sexual health and performance, which is beneficial whether your primary worry is low testosterone levels, erectile dysfunction, or the health of your prostate.

1. Spinach

Folate, which is found in abundance in spinach, is believed to improve blood flow. Folic acid is essential to the proper functioning of male sexual organs. Erectile dysfunction has been connected to folic acid levels that are too low in the blood. One cup (185 grams) of cooked spinach is equivalent to 77% of the Daily Value (DV) for folate, making it one of the foods with the highest folate content currently available.

Additionally, spinach has a respectable amount of magnesium, which not only contributes to the acceleration of blood flow but also has the potential to raise testosterone levels.

2. Cafeteria

According to the findings of a study that included more than 3,000 men, those who self-reported having the highest daily caffeine intake (85–300 mg per day, which is equivalent to 1–3 cups or 240–720 ml of coffee) had a lower risk of reporting erectile dysfunction than those who had the lowest caffeine intake. This was found to be the case regardless of the amount of coffee consumed.

3. Apples

One of the less well-known advantages of apples pertains to the health of the prostate, but they do have several positive effects on overall health.

The peels of apples, in particular, are rich sources of the bioactive chemical known as ursolic acid. According to the findings of one study conducted in test tubes, ursolic acid has the potential to "starve" prostate cancer cells and stop their growth. Note, however, that a great deal more research is required to properly understand how this effect might translate to eating apple peels rather than directly applying ursolic acid to cancer cells.

In any case, the results of previous research point to the fact that men who eat a diet rich in fruits and vegetables have a better chance of surviving prostate cancer.

4. Avocados

When the avocado was first discovered by the Aztecs around 500 B.C.E., they gave it the name of a word that meant "testicles" because of its shape and the fact that it grows in pairs on avocado trees.

Avocados are loaded with vitamin E, which research suggests may enhance the quality of sperm in men who struggle with infertility. There is 21% of the daily value for vitamin E in a single medium-sized (150-gram) avocado. Zinc is a vital mineral that plays role in the creation of testosterone, the quality of sperm, and fertility. One medium-sized avocado (150 grams) offers 9% of the daily need for zinc.

5. Chili peppers

Are you able to withstand the intensity? One study indicated that men who favored spicy food had higher amounts of testosterone in their saliva compared to guys who chose food with milder flavors.

Although this does not indicate that eating spicy food can enhance testosterone levels, the chemical capsaicin, which is contained in hot peppers, may have some advantages in the bedroom.

Intake of capsaicin through food can trigger pleasure regions in the brain, which in turn has the potential to increase mood and give an aphrodisiac effect. However, the majority of the study regarding capsaicin and mood has been done in animal experiments; as a result, the findings should be interpreted with some level of caution.

6. Carrots

Do you want to increase the number of sperm you produce? According to research, you should consume more carrots. In traditional medical practice, they have also been advised for a long time to treat male infertility. Due to the high carotenoid content of this vegetable, there is a possibility that both sperm count and motility (the movement and swimming of sperm) would improve. Carrots include carotenoids, which are orange-pigmented antioxidants that are responsible for many of the carrot's health advantages.

Dr. John K. Moore

7. Oats

Although oatmeal is not the first item that springs to mind when one thinks of sexual health, there is some evidence to suggest that eating oatmeal may have a positive impact.

Tomatoes, which are rich in both nutrients and antioxidants, may have various positive effects on male reproductive and sexual health, as well as on the health of the prostate.

They are rich in lycopene, an antioxidant that is characterized by their red color and has been associated with improved sperm production. In addition, they have a high

vitamin C content, which research suggests may be associated with enhanced sperm counts in men who are otherwise healthy.

Consumption of tomatoes, which are rich in the antioxidant lycopene, may also be connected with a reduced chance of developing prostate cancer.

In conclusion, one underpowered study involving 44 men who struggled with infertility found that males who drank tomato juice daily for 12 weeks had better sperm and greater motility in their sperm.

The bare essentials

Although there is some evidence suggesting that these eight foods have favorable benefits on male fertility, sexual health, or prostate health, the majority of the research in this area is inconclusive.

One thing to keep in mind, however, is that each of these meals is entire and has had only a small amount of processing.

It has been demonstrated that dietary patterns that are abundant in fruits, vegetables, whole grains, and other foods that are minimally processed, along with an adequate amount of protein and healthy fats, can help reduce the risk of erectile dysfunction, improve prostate health, and maximize fertility.

Dr. John K. Moore

Chapter 3

Surgical Penile Enlargement

What is penis enlargement surgery?

Surgery that makes your penis appear to be larger is known as penile augmentation surgery. Surgery is just one of the many ways that people could attempt to achieve this goal.

There are a variety of methods that can be used to increase the size of your penis, including the following: a surgical procedure designed to lengthen your penis (increase its length). A surgical procedure that enlarges your penis (increases its girth or circumference around the shaft). Liposuction reduces the size of your stomach to give the appearance of having a larger penis.

Who needs to have surgery to have their penis enlarged?

If you have a micropenis or your penis is buried, there may be medical reasons for you to consider having your penis enlarged surgically.

Congenital conditions are ones that you are born with, and having a micropenis, often known as a very little penis, is one of those conditions. The term "buried penis" refers to a penis that is hidden behind the skin from view from the scrotum, stomach, or thighs. This can be present at birth, but it can also develop later in life.

To restore a functional penis, these issues frequently lead patients to seek surgical intervention. These functions consist of the following:

- Having the ability to urinate while standing.
- Being capable of having sexual encounters that are deeply intimate

Who else besides these people would be interested in having their penises surgically enlarged?

The majority of the time, however, people who are interested in penile enlargement surgery aren't happy with the way their penis looks in its natural state.

Even when they can have penetrative intercourse or urinate while standing, they are nonetheless concerned that their penis isn't long enough or wide enough. They might believe that neither the length nor the girth is sufficient for the job.

The majority of people have penises that can perform what the penis was designed to do, which is to engage in sexual activity as well as urinate (pee) standing up. This is the primary reason why this issue is mostly one of perception. Some people have persistent and irritating concerns about the size of their penis, which can influence their day-to-day existence. While many people do occasionally wonder if the size of their penis is normal, other people do so just infrequently (their work, their relationships, and their overall mood).

If you are concerned about the size of your penis and find that it is having a negative impact on your life, even though a medical professional has assured you that the size of your penis is normal, you may be suffering from a condition known as penile dysmorphophobia disorder (PDD) or small penis anxiety.

A kind of body dysmorphic illness known as PDD (Penile Dysmorphophobia Disorder) has been described. PDD sufferers have the mistaken belief that their own penises are smaller than they are, while they also have the misconception that the penises of other people are larger than they are. PDD can put a person in a depressive state and can make it difficult to have an erection.

One type of worry is called SPA, which stands for "small penis anxiety." People who have SPA are more likely to have anxiety in settings where another person may have the opportunity to see their genitals, such as in a locker room or while engaging in sexual activity, since they are concerned that their penis is smaller than what is considered normal.

What may one expect during the process of having their penis enlarged?

Increasing the size of a man's penises can be accomplished through a variety of surgical methods. There are, however, very few procedures that operate consistently well to increase penile size or length. These treatments are quite rare.

When creating marketing brochures, companies frequently employ deceptive "before and after" photographs in the hope of attracting potential customers. Procedures such as these are frequently carried out:

Ligamentolysis is a surgical procedure that involves cutting the suspensory ligament that links your penis to your pubic bone. The penis seems to be longer and hangs lower when it is flaccid. Penis enlargement by the use of autologous fat involves the removal of fat from your body through liposuction by a medical professional, who then injects the fat into your penis to enhance its circumference.

Penis augmentation with dermal fillers is the injection of cosmetic fillers under the skin of the penis by a medical professional (subcutaneously). Some of these are far less hazardous than others.

Surgical excision of the suprapubic fat pad In males who have a penis that seems to be "buried," the fatty tissue that surrounds the penis may be surgically removed.

This does not result in an increase in the size of your penis; rather, it decreases the size of the tissues that surround it, so revealing the actual length of the penis.

What happens after penis enlargement?

When you are about to go from the office or the operating facility, your physician will provide you with instructions. The kind of treatment you received will determine how long you have to stay home from work or school and how long you have to wait before you can engage in sexual activity again after the procedure. This may take as long as six weeks after some of the more intrusive operations.

Chapter 4

Penile Enlargement Without Involving Surgery

A significant advance in penile enlargement has been made possible by recent technological advances in dermal fillers. To considerably increase the girth and width of the penis, the same products that are FDA allowed to augment cheeks and chins are injected into the penile shaft and head. This creates the appearance of a significantly larger penis.

In terms of both aesthetics and intimate connections, the most desirable quality is girth. Injections designed to enhance the penis have the most significant impact on the girth or width of the penis. Recent research conducted at the University of Texas found that the majority of male partners (90%) would rather have an increase in their penile girth (wide) than an increase in their penile length.

Fillers for the genital area function in a manner not dissimilar to that of fillers for the face in that they add volume where it is lacking. This therapy for an enlarged penile can enhance the girth and improve the overall appearance of the genital area. It is administered by injecting a solution directly into the penis. Penile enhancement using dermal fillers can, in essence, provide men with a significant confidence boost and help them feel more at ease in their own skin by increasing the size of their testicles.

The treatment to enlarge the penile size is done under local anesthetic and takes approximately half an hour to complete. In the majority of instances, the microcannula approach is utilized, and just two injection sites are utilized. When compared to several injections with sharp needles, microcannulas provide a higher level of safety and reduce the risk of bruising.

Patients see an instant improvement, which then continues for another two to four weeks. The goods that were utilized in the treatment will determine how long the outcomes will last. Following the operation, patients may experience mild to moderate transient edema as well as the possibility of bruising. In most circumstances, sexual activity can be resumed between five and seven days after treatment.

The goods that were utilized in the treatment will determine how long the outcomes will last. Voluma XC is the product that has been shown to be the most successful and durable. When using Voluma XC for penile enlargement, between 5 and 15 syringes must be injected into the penile shaft and glans (head). When doing penis enlargement with Voluma XC, we are able to give bulk savings on the price per syringe due to the product's popularity.

The base treatment consists of five syringes of the product of your choice; the pricing for this is listed below. Patients have the option of purchasing more syringes on the same day as their treatment at a substantial cost saving.

What exactly does the process entail?

Fillers made of hyaluronic acid (HA) create exceptional girth enlargement and resistance to external compression; this gives the penis a natural sensation whether it is flaccid or erect. The results are long-lasting and have an aesthetic aspect that is really gratifying. Injectable fillers made of hyaluronic acid are favored since the substance may be quickly eliminated if it ever becomes necessary to do so.

A topical anesthetic cream was applied to the penis. After that, a micro cannula is utilized to do a gradual injection of the hyaluronic acid filler just below the superficial layer of the dermis. Because the fillers all include lidocaine, the patient will have far less pain and suffering throughout the process.

This is a process that may be completed in less than an hour and takes place in an office setting. After the surgery, the patient can immediately return to their regular routine without any restrictions.

Chapter 5

How to Increase the Size of Your Penis

1.Penis enlargement strategies or approaches couldn't give you identical results. According to the different kinds of procedures and items that are available on the worldwide health market, such as creams, stretchers, pumps, weight extenders, and Bio Magnify Pills, amongst other things. A love connection can quickly become strained if the two people involved have interactions with a common acquaintance that are unproductive or dull. Learning new methods to pleasure a lady is essential to securing her affection and maintaining a healthy level of sexual desire between the two of you. The manner of solar light can always be used to discover useful hints and recommendations on how to stimulate her. In this way, you will have the opportunity to give your wife an experience that will rank among the most memorable of her entire life.

The use of natural male enhancement procedures can increase your size by as much as 3 feet in length and 1 foot in girth, depending on how much you want to change it. I escaped from a house that was quite poor. 5 inches in length and 5 inches in circumference to over 8 inches in length and just 6 inches in circumference. Bio Magnify Male Enhancement Here is all you need to know about natural ways to increase the size of your male organ so that you may use your hands to grow by at least three feet.

2. Costs: the price of male enhancement creams might range widely. As is the case with the majority of products, Bio Magnify Pills may come in both pricey and more affordable varieties. Nevertheless, regardless of which path you take, there will inevitably be a cost involved. It is true that if you plan and put into action a well-thought-out social media strategy, it may pay off in the form of cash. You'll be able to count on a steady flow of qualified customers who can't wait to buy what you're selling or test out what you're offering.

Are you finally prepared to buy any woman a body-quivering several times during the course of a single sitting? If you want to increase your chances of getting hired, lie about the simple fact that most men struggle to provide their partners with even a single child of various types. Have you ever considered the possibility that maintaining a higher standard is a form of competition among businesses?

It would appear that whoever possesses the larger is the more dominating party. The fact that women find those with more significance to be more attractive is one reason why men want to appear to have more of it.

It is not a well-kept secret that in today's environment, men's sexuality is receiving more attention than it ever has in the past. This is true of both women and men. A focus is being placed on operation, and a significant number of men are becoming progressively dissatisfied with their strength. Up until quite recently, there were very few available choices. Numerous guys are in a position to extend their lives for a number of years thanks to male enhancement products that are made from natural ingredients.

If you are intent on locating the most efficient method to acquire a bigger truth, you should ask this inquiry yourself. How effective are male enlargement Bio Magnify Pills? However, it is the method of enlargement that receives the most publicity, so it must be effective, right? The better reading is actually a before aid to make a decision on which approach is most effective.

The most effective male enhancement drug has enjoyed widespread acceptance for many years. Discover the 100% natural pill that has been used by a huge number of men in an effort to increase their size. If you are anything like the other 99% of men, you want to help you last longer in bed and deliver the best to your girlfriend. It might either help a person get rid of their lady or make their woman more receptive to their efforts to please their woman. You might be shocked to learn that there are only three stages involved in doing that.

This tried and true method requires roughly six minutes to carry out each Bio Magnify Pill every day over the course of a few months.

Many of the guys who have tried the method have witnessed advances in the length of their beards which can range from one to four inches in a period of six to eight weeks.

Dr. John K. Moore

We would be grateful if you could a few moments after you have finished reading, to please leave us a pleasing review on Amazon. Your review will help us to reach a wider audience and also help other readers to discover how helpful this book is.

Your time is valued as you are willing to share your thoughts.

Thank you in anticipation for the kind review.

Chapter 6

Best sex pills for men

Men in today's society frequently have issues such as low libido, erections that last for a limited amount of time, and premature ejaculation.

Sex is not only a part of a successful relationship (and an essential one), but it can also offer a multitude of health benefits, such as helping to burn calories, relieving stress, anxiety, and depression, lowering blood pressure, and even improving cardiovascular health. Sex is not only a part of a successful relationship (and an essential one). That is the reason why one could feel the urge to take male enhancement pills in their day-to-day existence.

When sexual performance concerns such as poor sex drive, erectile dysfunction, short-term erection, or premature ejaculation prevent a person from having a satisfying experience with their partner during sexual activity, nothing seems to be quite right.

Your physical and mental health are both severely impacted, not to mention the potential strain that is placed on the relationship you have with your partner.

Taking decisive action while there is still time is almost always the best course of action to adopt. You might want to begin by looking at some natural cures. We are discussing male enhancement pills that are derived from natural sources and may assist in improving the natural capabilities of the human body without exposing the body to any of the negative consequences that are typically linked with the consumption of pharmaceutical pharmaceuticals.

The majority of the male enhancement pill options that are currently available will be compared to a select few male enhancement supplements that we think to be both safe and considerably more effective than the majority of the male enhancement pill options currently available.

Also covered in this article will be a discussion of some of the most important considerations you should make before making any purchases of this kind from an online retailer.

1. Performer8 is ranked number one as the best male enhancement pill overall.

It is possible for Performer8 to increase a man's sexual performance by a factor of eight. Its formulation is made up of substances that are 100% natural, herbal, devoid of soy and gluten, and does not include any GMOs. In addition to giving firmer erections, higher semen density, quantity, and mobility, one may notice a boost in libido, sexual energy, and stamina.

- *Ingredients*

A potent combination of Muira Puama extract, KSM-66 Ashwagandha, ferrous bis-glycinate (an easily digestible type of iron), Maca root extract, Panax Ginseng, Barrenwort (Horny Goat Weed), Pine Bark extract, Glucuronolactone, and grape seed extract are contained within this dietary supplement.

- *Dosage*

Consume daily with a meal, three capsules in total.

- *Highlights*

Nine components that are entirely natural

Non-genetically modified and vegan-friendly.

Free of soy and gluten and with an easy dosage

No artificial additives

2. VigRX Plus Is a Sexual Enhancement Supplement That Helps Treat Erectile Dysfunction

In addition to increasing the frequency and intensity of orgasms with more controlled ejaculations, VigRX Plus may increase the hardness and duration of erections. When you use VigRX Plus, you can anticipate experiencing increased sexual stamina and vitality in addition to a bigger, deeper penis and greater penetration.

In addition to promoting better blood circulation, this formulation may also assist boost your mood and maintain mental equilibrium by lowering levels of tension and worry.

Components The components of this clinically researched and developed supplement include Damiana, Epimedium leaf extract, Asian Red Ginseng, Muira Pauma bark extract, Hawthorn berry, Catuaba bark extract, Saw Palmetto, Ginkgo Biloba, and Bioperine®. Other components include Catuaba bark extract, Hawthorn berry, and Muira Pauma bark extract (piperine from black pepper).

3. TestoPrime: The Most Effective Pills to Boost Sexual Drive.

TestoPrime is a potent testosterone booster that is made entirely of natural components and is suitable for vegans. It does not contain any soy, dairy, or gluten products and does not contain any soy. It is possible that it may assist in naturally elevated levels of free testosterone in the body, which will result in improved desire, erection, and ejaculation.

- *Ingredients*

D-Aspartic acid, Panax Ginseng, KSM-66® Ashwagandha extract, Fenugreek, green tea extract (70% Catechins), Pomegranate extract (ellagic acid), Zinc, and Vitamin D,

Vitamins B5, and B6, black pepper extract, and garlic extract are all included in this supplement.

- *Dosage*

Four TestoPrime capsules should be taken first thing in the morning (preferably with breakfast).

4. Male Extra - Pills for Improving the Size of Your Erections

In addition to enhancing sexual prowess, Male Extra can also improve blood flow to the penis, which can lead to longer-lasting performance and enjoyment during sexual encounters. For the highest possible level of performance enhancement, take this supplement, which is made up entirely of all-natural, risk-free substances.

- *Highlights*

Ingredients that are 100% natural and risk-free

Unique formula

No artificial additives

The recommended daily dosage is three capsules, to be taken with a meal.

Appropriate for use by any and all guys.

5. ProSolution Plus, a Male Sexual Enhancement Supplement
The most effective treatment available for premature ejaculation is found in ProSolution Plus. Along with improved sexual drive, energy levels, and sexual endurance, one can anticipate having better control over one's ejaculations after using this supplement. Additionally, one can anticipate having a higher sex drive.
Ingredients in ProSolution Plus are 100% natural, non-toxic, and clinically proven to be effective.

Components All-natural ingredients, including:
Tribulus Terrestris, Withania somnifera, Asparagus ascendens, Mucuna pruriens, Asteracantha longifolia, Curculigo orchioides, and Asphaltum. Ingredients

6. Max Performer: Powerful Pills for Enhancing Penis Size and Sexual Arousal: The male enhancement pills sold under the brand name Max Performer have the potential to boost a man's self-esteem and improve his sexual performance by boosting orgasms and providing him with longer, harder erections.

The supplement known as Max Performer is made entirely from natural, risk-free substances that are known for their powerful effects.

7. Semenax, Pills for Penis Enlargement That Help You Ejaculate Better: Semenax is a product for men's sexual health that has been shown to increase the volume of sperm and create orgasms that are both longer and more powerful. This indicates that a person taking Semenax will be able to deliver the greatest amount of pleasure and volume of sperm to his partner.

The chemicals in Semanax are completely natural and have been shown to be effective in clinical trials.

- *Ingredients include:*

Swedish flower pollen, L-Arginine HCL, L-Lysine, Epimedium Sagittatum (also known as horny goat weed), Zinc Aspartate, L-Carnitine, Catuaba Bark, Pumpkin Seed (Zinc Oxide), Maca, Vitamin E, Pine Bark extract, Muira Puama, Hawthorn, Cranberry extract, Sarsaparilla, Avena Sativa extract, and Butea Super.

- *Dosage*

Take four capsules once every 24 hours with any meal.

How and Why Were These Male Enhancement Pills Chosen?

The composition of male enhancement tablets might vary greatly from brand to brand. There are some that are more efficient than others, while others have absolutely no effect at all. Still, others have the potential to contribute nothing positive to the human body and may even be harmful.

As a customer, you need to be careful of deceptive advertising practices and make choices that are in your best interest, because every other company in the industry has the same goal of making its mark on the market. Always make sure you're a savvy shopper. If some fundamental guidelines are adhered to, the challenge is significantly reduced.

One must be aware of the fact that these dietary supplements are not capable of totally curing any significant medical issue that requires the assistance of a medical professional (nor do the manufacturers claim that they are!).

If you are suffering from a serious medical issue, taking these pills will not provide you with a long-term solution to your problem. On the other hand, you might find that using them frequently and persistently helps, provided that you do so under the supervision of a medical professional. The fact that these pills do not provide any significant risks to one's health is easily the best aspect of them.

It is important to keep in mind that falling prey to companies that offer fraudulent or low-quality medications is not only a waste of money; it can utterly destroy any hope of saving your connection with your life partner.

During the course of investigating the most popular brands of male health supplements, we looked into a variety of aspects and characteristics that lend these tablets their suitability for ongoing use. Since the benefits of using these naturally enhanced performance substances on a regular and consistent basis are not immediately apparent, we made sure that purchasing these products would be a worthwhile investment for those looking to improve their sexual lives.

Considerations to Keep in Mind When Choosing a Male Enhancement Method

1. Composition of the Product When it comes to introducing the body to something novel, the composition of the product is the single most crucial component. Because these products need to be consumed on a daily basis, it is in your best interest to have a comprehensive understanding of the components and the effects that they can have. We went to great lengths to ensure that these products include nothing but natural, unadulterated extracts that are free from any harmful substances.

In addition to this, we made sure that there were no artificial ingredients of any kind, which could be harmful to your health (or pocket). It's possible that adding fillers that aren't necessary will make an otherwise effective combination of substances less effective overall.

2. The efficiency of it: Even if some natural extracts could have a beneficial effect on you, taking a supplement that has a bunch of the same elements might not be the best idea.

In order for any mixture of natural materials to be effective as a whole, each individual component of the mixture must be compatible with the other components of the mixture.

3. Dosage

It is crucial to make a conscious effort to take the medication at the appropriate time each day in order to achieve a gradual, safe, and smooth transition. That is also true for drugs designed to boost sexual performance in men. These natural pills are intended to progressively improve sexual function rather than dramatically increase it all of a sudden.

As a result, we made an effort to include companies that produce tablets that have the ideal quantities of their constituents and that may be taken in a convenient and consistent manner. The timing of our users as well as their frequency of it was a significant consideration in the decision-making process that we went through.

4. Reputation of the Brand

There are a variety of male enhancement pills on the market, and many of their particular brands are highly popular. And for a very excellent reason in particular. These pills have accomplished an excellent level of market penetration thanks to the superior quality of their products and the exceptional customer service they provide.

It is not worth either the money or the time to invest in brands that do not make the effort to correctly direct their clients along the path they are traveling.

In order to verify the total efficacy of these pills, we read the reviews, carried out surveys, and even consulted with professionals and specialists in the field of medicine.

Dr. John K. Moore

We would be grateful if you could a few moments after you have finished reading, to please leave us a pleasing review on Amazon. Your review will help us to reach a wider audience and also help other readers to discover how helpful this book is.

Your time is valued as you are willing to share your thoughts.

Thank you in anticipation for the kind review.

Chapter 6

Penis Stretching Device

The PHALLOSAN forte

Phallosan forte is worldwide the only patented orthopedic belt system with a new, breakthrough vacuum protection technology - the even faster route to penis growth or straightening, helping you to attain new confidence and an enhanced quality of life.

Phallosan forte also enlarges the glans, as the vacuum surrounds the whole penis. Most other devices start with tension behind the glans. We have 18 years of experience in the production and implementation of technologies for penile growth, penis lengthening, and/or penis straightening. Years of study and the evaluation of thousands of client reactions have helped us design and refine the phallosan forte System. Phallosan forte satisfies all medical regulations and holds the CE symbol to confirm it.

There are "stretchers" and there is a phallosan forte. Learn more about how our vacuum protector system with soft power works:

The principle

Stretching the penile tissue continuously and gently encourages the formation of new cells. Phallosan forte operates on the entire penis, beginning with the glans, by generating an extremely imperceptible vacuum. The PHALLOSAN forte's excellent level of comfort makes it simple for the user to wear the system for ten hours straight without experiencing any discomfort at all—a crucial requirement for success! Phallosan forte saves you embarrassment because our method never causes your pants to come undone like other systems.

If used properly, phallosan forte use is painless. As the system on the penis shaft can adjust at any time to a potential erection, the phallosan forte can also be worn at night. It doesn't prevent blood flow. Injury risks don't exist like they do with other systems.

The CE emblem appears on the phallosan forte, and it complies with EC Council Directive 93/42/EEC. Additionally, it complies with EN 980, EN ISO 14971, and EN ISO 10993-1 standards. It is produced in accordance with medical specifications established by European health authorities. The materials needed for manufacturing have undergone biocompatibility testing and are well tolerated. Formaldehyde is absent from the cloth stretch belt designed specifically for PHALLOSAN forte penis growth. The sleeves are latex- and allergen-free. Medical foam silicone has been specifically chosen to make the counter support for the textile stretch belt application that's painless and natural.

The device has outcomes that can be seen after being worn painlessly for up to 12 hours each day or night. The glans grow significantly while being kept from slipping out by the vacuum (negative pressure) in the suction bell. The belt tension can be changed indefinitely.

The parts are simple to clean. There are comprehensive, illustrated use instructions included. The belt's components can all be ordered separately. Replacement is simple and convenient with velcro fasteners.

If the suction is too powerful, the newly created protection cap prevents swelling and redness of the foreskin and glans. Similar to a compression stocking or a jet pilot's pressurized gear, it applies gentle pressure to the skin's surface tissue. Now that the pressure has been raised, success can come even faster.

Chapter 7

Permanent Male Enhancement

The "Permanent Dermal Filler Injection Technique," also known as a penile enlargement employing a collagen layering activation filler treatment, is generally utilized for circumferential or girth expansion of the penis. This technique involves the use of new and unique materials (this technique is also used for Scrotal Skin enhancement and reconstruction). This expansion has an effect on the penis, the glans, and the scrotum when they are in both the flaccid and erect stages. Despite the fact that length gains have been observed, this has not been the case for each and every patient.

1. A local anesthetic cream is applied to the vaginal region to numb it.

2. Once the affected region has been completely numbed, the doctor will be able to start the process of repeated microinjections by making use of a needle with a small caliber.

3. The physician is able to work on the entire region, artistically sculpting the penile shaft, the glans, and the scrotum according to the procedure plan for the patient. Please take note that one of the various fillers that can be utilized is the Silikon 1000 (or another similar product), which can be seen above.

4. Following the injection of the filler material into the skin layers of the penile shaft, the penis will become larger, and the body will now start to react to the filler formula by producing new collagen. Collagen is a type of protein that accounts for a significant portion of the composition of connective tissues in general as well as the skin.

5. A specialized wrap is then applied around the area surrounding the penis.

Penile wraps are used as a help to assist in shaping the newly formed collagen to provide a more symmetrical and even shape to the penile shaft. These penile wraps are used as an aid to assist in molding the newly formed collagen.

After the enhancement procedure, which takes about an hour to complete, the penile shaft will be wrapped with gauze, stretch wrap, and a few other elements – as seen in the photo above – and the patient will leave the office in this fashion.

The enhancement procedure is intended to increase the size of the patient's penile erection. A number of re-wrappings will have to be performed over the course of the subsequent 35 days of recovery. The primary purpose of these re-wrappings is to monitor the healing process and adapt the post-procedure recovery process to the specific requirements of the patient, in addition to ensuring that the genital region is kept clean.

After around 35 days have passed since the procedure, one can observe the results. The majority of the outcomes can be observed in approximately four weeks or less, despite the fact that there is a possibility that some collagen production may continue to take place for as long as ninety days. It is possible to undergo a second operation or any other procedure that follows the first one as soon as five weeks (or 35 days) have passed after the first one. Men who know they want at least a significant increase in circumference, who have a specific goal in mind, or who, after experiencing the benefits of the male enhancement procedure, desire to continue enjoying the added increase in gains until they are satisfied should consider having a second procedure. There are virtually no restrictions placed on the number of procedures that a patient may undergo.

After the initial surgery, the patient will have to wait around five weeks before they may undergo any additional treatments, including the second procedure. After the first treatment, it is normal for 90% of patients to gain between 3/4 and 1 inch, which is the predicted result, and then they will gain an additional 3/4 to 1 inch on the second treatment. Depending on how quickly and effectively the patient recovers from the prior treatment, those patients who seek girth gains of more than 2 inches will typically require a third surgery. The number of procedures required to get the desired results can be repeated, if desired.